Yoga Ba:

A Beginner's Guide to Yoga Poses, Exercises and Techniques to Relieve Stress, Improve Flexibility and Strengthen Mind, Body and Spirit

By Matt McKinney

Contents

Thank you for buying this book and I hope that you will find it useful. If you will want to share your thoughts on this book, you can do so by leaving a review on the Amazon page, it helps me out a lot.

Introduction

As we head into this intense brand-new millennium, we're continuously reminded of the blend of west and east. Whether it's via satellite tv which beams in creations from various cultures, taking pleasure in music and books from far-off lands which, just a generation or two back, could not be accessed, and-- obviously-- interacting with individuals throughout space and time via the Web and other telecommunications innovations, the world has actually ended up being a much tinier location. Undoubtedly, when Marshall McLuhan mentioned the term Global Village, even he most likely didn't imagine so much, so quickly, so soon.

Riding the trend of information which now crisscrosses our small world is a thing which has its roots in old history, yet is experiencing a blossoming in the west which keeps on getting momentum with every year that passes. Whether it's at a regional YMCA or a lavish spiritual retreat in the Everglades, Yoga is developing itself as a pillar in western culture.

Nevertheless, lots of people hesitate to experience the physical, psychological, and mental health advantages of yoga; and there is actually only one significant reason for this: false information.

While many individuals may really delight in yoga and find it to be the side-effect free answer to a great deal of their psychological and physical disorders, they simply do not understand enough about the topic to take that initial step.

In addition, a stereotype out there that appears to continue in spite of proof to the contrary is that yoga is a religious following; and that to feel its numerous health advantages in some way obliges one to renounce their faith or, even worse, flee to some commune and consume tofu in between chanting sessions.

While, certainly, if you wish to head to a retreat and take pleasure in chanting and tofu, that's most likely feasible (nearly anything is feasible, as long as it's legal and individuals wish to do it, right?).

Yet that image of yoga-- individuals with shaved heads and giving flowers to complete strangers at the airport-- is, in no way, the general picture. Yoga is actually an extremely basic, available, and in numerous nations around the globe, regular thing to do.

In that light, this book is produced with one objective in mind: to debunk yoga for you, and supply you with a clear, basic, and enjoyable intro to the subject.

If you have actually never ever been exposed to any type of yoga (except for what you may have seen on tv), then this book is for you!

Additionally, even if you have actually experienced some sort of yoga (possibly a buddy dragged you to a class at the neighborhood recreation center years back), this book is going to rekindle your interest in the subject and reconnect you to a mode of mind focus and body movement which has actually resided in ancient lands for thousand years.

This guide is arranged into 5 sections:

I. What is Yoga

II. Benefits of Yoga?

III. Various Types of Yoga

IV. Yoga Poses For Beginners

V. Accessories and Equipment

As you go through these parts, please remember that there is definitely no intention here, indirectly or directly to promote or endorse any religious view. This is due to the fact that the view of this guide is the identical view which is held by the world's primary yoga authorities: that it is not a religion. It does not have a dogma.

While there are undoubtedly various streams and schools of yoga-- there are in fact hundreds of them-- they have actually all managed to exist side-by-side rather comfortably since, mainly, yoga is not evangelical, which just implies that it does not look to spread itself as part of its objective.

Please keep in mind that the declaration above in no way slams or talks about evangelical orders; the point here is just that the large bulk of yoga movements do not see spreading out yoga as a tenet of its identity.

Yet, as the yoga which is explained in this book (and experienced in the majority of the globe) is not a religion, it does really effortlessly fit into numerous individuals' current religious system.

To put it simply, if you are a Catholic, a Muslim, a Protestant, a Sikh, a Jew, or any other thing and identify yourself as a part of any faith whatsoever, yoga does not ask you to substitute that faith with something else, or provide you a contradictory or contending view of what you currently believe.

So please keep in mind: yoga, as it is talked about in this guide, is not a religion.

As we'll start to comprehend in the following part of this guide, yoga is actually absolutely nothing more, and absolutely nothing less, than using the power of human attention, and utilizing it to aid the mind and body. It is a way of living, in the moment.

Chapter 1: What is Yoga?

Yoga may appear as a complex concept; or, at the minimum, a dizzying range of physical tricks which turn apparently happy-looking humans into pretzels.

Or perhaps more perplexing, as we have mentioned in the beginning, a stereotype does exist somewhere, where the term yoga is associated with the cult, or some type of antiquated spiritual belief which obliges one to sell their home, quit their job, and go reside in the middle of nowhere.

In reality, Yoga is an extremely standard thing; and if you have actually had the chance to go to a nation where it has actually been established for generations-- India, China, Japan, and others-- it's truly rather, well, common.

The yoga practice arrived to the west back in 1893 when one of India's popular gurus, Swami Vivekananda, was welcomed at the World Fair in

Chicago. He is currently recognized for having stimulated the West's yoga interest.

Actually, the term yoga originates from the Sanskrit word Yug, which means: "to yoke, join, bind, or direct one's attention." Simultaneously, yoga can likewise indicate ideas like union, fusion, and discipline.

The sacred Hindu scriptures (an old Indian belief system with a worldwide presence) likewise specify yoga as "unitive discipline"; the sort of discipline which, based upon specialists Stephan Bodian and Georg Feuerstein in their book Living Yoga, results in an inner and external union, happiness and harmony.

Essentially, yoga is most typically recognized as mindful living; of using one's inside potential for joy (what Sankrit calls Ananda).

What Yoga Is not

Often it's useful to comprehend things by what they aren't; specifically, when handling a subject such as Yoga, that is rather quickly misconstrued.

Yoga scholars and authors Bodian and Feuerstein aid us comprehend yoga by informing us what it is not:

Yoga is not calisthenics. While it holds true that yoga entails numerous postures-- specifically in hatha yoga-- these are just meant to make individuals connect with their internal feelings.

Yoga is not a meditation system-- or a religion-- the way lots of people are misguided to think. Meditation is just part of the entire procedure of bringing ourselves into the spiritual world.

The Core of Yoga

Practically all yogic philosophy and science claims that a human is but a piece of a massive universe, and when this person finds out how to commune with this greatness, then that person obtains union with a thing which is larger than that person. This attachment or tapping into anything larger, therefore, allows one to walk the real path of joy. By streaming together with the force, the person has the ability to find reality.

And with reality comes awareness; however, to achieve awareness, our words, ideas and deeds need to be based upon reality. Individuals go to yoga courses and head to studios to discover brand-new methods in yoga.

Physical Health and Yoga

Yoga does not see a difference between the mind and the body, and this is a comprehension which western psychology has actually had for several years now (the connection between physical and psychological health, and vice versa).

If you have actually come to this guide aiming to comprehend yoga as a way to aid your body recover, then do not worry; you have actually come to the appropriate place!

Yoga is undoubtedly a procedure that includes discharging obstructed stress and energy in the body and aiding to make the muscles, joints, tendons, ligaments, and all other parts work to their highest capacity.

Yogis believe that humans are perfectly created, by nature, to be versatile and nimble; and tightness and absence of mobility just show up when the body out of alignment or unhealthy.

For that reason, numerous individuals have actually found themselves in a yoga class, in the hopes of enhancing their physical health; and maybe you might be among them. If that holds true, then carry on reading!

There are tested physical advantages of yoga, that involve:

More range of motion and flexibility

Lowered pain in muscles and joints

More powerful immunity

More powerful lung capacity and for that reason better respiration

Boosted metabolism (which could result in weight reduction!).

Better sleep (specifically because of better breathing and a more oxygenated body).

Given that specific yoga practices need poses to be mastered, yoga has actually constantly assisted to promote the body's flexibility; it likewise assists in lubricating the joints, tendons and ligaments. Yoga cleanses by boosting the circulation of blood to different body parts. It assists to tone and revitalize the muscles which have actually grown weak and limp.

So please do remember that, while yoga is typically talked about in regards to its psychological approach, there are clear and tested physical advantages which are a part of this approach.

For that reason, if weight reduction is your objective, or the capability to shovel the snow in winter season without your back hurting for days, then yoga is as practical a choice to you as it is for the stressed-out business executive who has to discover a method for dealing with the madness in her hectic life!

Chapter 2: Why is Yoga Good?

As we have actually repeatedly mentioned in this guide, yoga is not a religion. It may be if one desires it to be, and it could co-exist with a current religion. However, yoga itself is not religious in a way that it concentrates on faith or belief.

Yoga is a science; and undoubtedly, in lots of locations worldwide (such as India), it is described as a science. This is not just wordplay; it genuinely is seen as a science, which indicates that it is comprehended in regards to the scientific method.

Yogic science aims to validate cause and effect and construct concepts based upon unbiased observations. Certainly, in lots of locations on the planet, to be a yogic master of any trustworthiness, one needs to be extremely informed in the sciences, consisting of biological sciences and the physics.

This conversation on yoga as science is necessary for us to have here due to the fact that it permits us to smartly ask the question: what are the advantages of yoga? Besides, if yoga is a belief or a faith, then asking this question isn't reasonable; since it's one that yoga may not respond to in a way which we can objectively comprehend.

In the end, yoga is a science; as pragmatic and empirical as kinesiology, or exercise science, which wants to comprehend how the body acts and responds to modifications in the internal physical environment. Each of us has a right to ask the fundamental question such as why bother with yoga?

Certainly, while the experience of yoga may not be minimized to words-- just as reading a book on getting ready for a marathon will not, in fact, prepare you physically to participate a marathon-- the objectives and concepts of yoga can quickly be gone over.

Here's the Mayo Clinic's take on the meditation advantages:

Meditation is utilized by individuals who are completely healthy as a method of reducing stress. However, if you have a medical condition that's gotten worse by stress, you may discover the practice useful in lowering the stress-related impacts of allergic reactions, asthma, arthritis and chronic pain, to name a few.

Yoga includes a series of poses, throughout which you look at your breathing carefully. You could approach yoga as a method to promote physical versatility, endurance and strength or as a method to improve your spirituality.

Yoga Benefits

Yoga via meditation functions incredibly to attain harmony and it aids the mind to function in sync with the body. How frequently do we discover that we are not able to perform our activities effectively and in a gratifying way due to the confusion and disputes in our head weighing down greatly upon us?

Stress is the primary suspect impacting all aspects of our endocrinal, physical, and psychological systems. And with the aid of yoga, these things could be fixed.

At the physical level, yoga and its cleansing practices have actually shown to be exceptionally helpful for different conditions.

Listed beneath are simply a few of the advantages of yoga which you may get:

Advantage of Yoga no. 1: Yoga is understood to boost flexibility; yoga has poses which activate the various joints. Including those joints which are not acted upon with routine workout regimens.

Advantage of Yoga no. 2: Yoga likewise boosts the joint, tendon and ligament lubrication. The well-researched yoga poses work the various ligaments and tendons of the body. It has actually likewise been discovered that somebody who might begin doing yoga might experience rather amazing versatility on those body parts that have actually not been purposely worked upon.

Advantage of Yoga no. 3: yoga likewise massages all bodily organs. Yoga is maybe the only exercise which could work on through your internal organs in a comprehensive way, consisting of those which barely get stimulated externally throughout our whole lifetime.

Advantage of Yoga no. 4: Yoga acts in a wholesome way on the numerous body parts. This massage and stimulation of the organs, consequently, aids us by keeping away illness and offering a forewarning at the initial feasible example of a likely start of illness or condition. Among the significant advantages of yoga is the uncanny feeling of awareness which it establishes in the practitioner of an upcoming health condition or infection. This, consequently, makes it possible for the individual to take corrective, pre-emptive action.

Advantage of Yoga no. 5: yoga detoxifies the whole body. It carefully stretches the joints and muscles. While massaging the numerous organs, yoga guarantees the optimal blood supply to different body parts. This assists in the flushing out of toxins from each cranny and nook of your body in addition to offering nourishment up to the final point. This results in benefits like postponed aging, energy and an amazing enthusiasm for life.

Advantages of Yoga no. 6: yoga is, likewise, an exceptional method to tone your muscles. Muscles that have actually been limp and weak are stimulated consistently to shed excess flaccidity and fat.

However, these massive physical advantages are simply a "side effect" of this powerful practice. What yoga does is balancing the body with the mind, and these lead to genuine huge benefits.

It is well-known that the will of the mind has actually allowed individuals to accomplish remarkable physical accomplishments, which proves beyond doubt the connection between body and mind.

actually, yoga equates to meditation, due to the fact that both interact in accomplishing the common objective of the unity of body, mind, and spirit that can cause an experience of everlasting happiness which you may just feel via yoga.

The meditative practices via yoga aid in attaining a psychological balance via detachment.

This, consequently, develops an impressive peace and a favorable outlook, which likewise has remarkable advantages on the physical health.

The Mind-Body Connection

Yoga is focused on the mind-body harmony. This mind-body harmony is attained via 3 things:

I.Poses (asanas).

II.Appropriate breathing (pranayama).

III.Meditation.

Body and mind draw motivation and assistance from the mixed practices of asanas, meditation and breathing. As individuals age (to yogis, aging is an artificial condition), our bodies end up being vulnerable to poisons and toxins (triggered by environmental and bad dietary elements).

Yoga assists us via a cleansing procedure, turning our bodies into a well-oiled and well-integrated piece of machinery.

Physical Benefits.

By balancing these 3 principles, the advantages of yoga are obtained. And just what are these advantages? Based upon www.abc-of-yoga.com, these advantages consist of:

Central nerve system equilibrium

Reduction in pulse.

Respiratory and blood pressure rates.

Cardiovascular performance.

Gastrointestinal stabilization.

Increased breath-holding time.

Better dexterity abilities.

Better balance.

Better depth perception.

Better memory.

Mental Benefits.

As noted above, Yoga likewise provides a range of mental advantages; and in fact, this is an extremely typical reason why individuals start practicing it in the first place. Possibly the most regularly pointed out mental advantage of yoga is a better capability to handle stress. Yoga decreases a person's levels of anxiety, depression, and sleepiness; hence allowing him/her to concentrate on what's spiritual and essential: attaining balance and joy.

Supporting a Healthy Way Of Life

There is some extremely intriguing psychology behind this that students of western thinkers (e.g. Freud, Fromm, Jung, and so on) are going to find familiar and, certainly, rather logical.

When a person chooses to be pleased, something inside that individual activates; a sort of awareness or will emerges. This awareness starts to observe the jungle of unfavorable thoughts which are swimming continuously across the mind.

Instead of attacking every one of these ideas-- since that would be an endless battle!-- yoga merely recommends to the individual to view that battle; and through that viewing, the tension will reduce (due to the fact that it ends up being uncovered and hence unfed by the unobserving, unconscious mind!).

Simultaneously, as the person starts to decrease their inner negativity levels, subsequent outer unfavorable behaviors start to fall of their own accord; habits like extreme drinking, psychological overindulging, and taking part in habits that, eventually, cause suffering and unhappiness.

With this being stated, it would be an overstatement to indicate that practicing yoga is the simple method to, say, stop cigarette smoking, or to begin working out routinely. If that held true, yoga would be perfect! Yoga merely says that, based upon logical and scientific cause and effect relationships which have actually been observed for centuries, that when an individual starts to feel great within, they naturally have a tendency to act in ways which boost and promote this sensation of inner health.

As such, while cigarette smoking (for instance) is a dependency and the body is going to respond to the minimizing of addicting components like tobacco and tar (simply to name 2 of many!), yoga is going to assist the procedure. It is going to assist to offer the person with the strength and reasoning that they require so as to find that smoking really does not make them feel great.

Actually, once they begin observing how they feel, they'll see without a doubt that rather than feeling great, cigarette smoking really makes one feel rather bad within; it's more difficult to breathe, for one.

Now, this book isn't a book about stoping smoking, and if you have actually battled with stopping smoking, then please do not be angered by any of this; there is no effort here whatsoever to suggest that stopping smoking is simple, or just a question of self-control.

Scientists have actually shown that there is a real physical dependency that is in place, together with a psychological dependency that could be just as powerful; maybe even more powerful.

The point here is just to assist you in comprehending that yoga could aid an individual make mindful living choices which encourage healthy and delighted living. This could involve:

Giving up smoking

Minimizing excess drinking

Eating better

Getting extra sleep

Lowering tension at work (and everywhere else).

Promoting more beneficial relationships all around.

Please keep in mind: yoga does not guarantee anybody that these things are going to just occur overnight. At most, yoga is the light that reveals you how unpleasant things in the basement actually are; and when that light is on, it ends up being far more uncomplicated-- not to mention time effective and efficient -- to tidy things up!

Psychological Advantages

Yoga has actually likewise been hailed for its unique capcapability to aid individuals get rid of sensations of hostility and inner bitterness. Due to removing these harmful feelings, the doorway to self-actualization and self-acceptance opens.

Pain Management Advantages

Pain management is another advantage of yoga. Given that pain and chronic pain are conditions which impact everyone at some time, comprehending the positive connection between pain management and yoga may be indispensable.

It could likewise be economically valuable considering that the pain medication market is a multi-billion dollar market and many individuals, particularly as they age, discover that their insurance coverage or government coverage will not cover certain over the –counter and pharmaceutical pain relief meds.

Yoga is thought to decrease pain by assisting the brain's pain center in managing the gate-controlling system situated in the spine and the secretion of natural pain relievers in the body.

Breathing exercises utilized in yoga could likewise decrease pain. Due to the fact that muscles have a tendency to unwind when you breathe out, extending the time of exhalation could aid to bring about relaxation and lower stress.

Awareness of breathing assists in attaining slower, calmer respiration and helps in pain management and relaxation. Yoga's addition of relaxation methods and meditation could likewise help in reducing pain. Part of the usefulness of yoga in minimizing pain is because of its focus on self-awareness.

This self-awareness could have a protective impact and make early prevention possible.

Chapter 3: Various Types Of Yoga

It's amusing to look at it in this manner. However, one of the important things which has actually promoted the yoga spreadin the west is the identical thing which can often stop somebody from really exploring it and for that reason experiencing its health advantages. This thing is variety.

In some cases when there is just one of something-- like one language, or one idea, or one anything-- it's tough for that thing to spread out beyond those who follow it, agree with it, or merely want it to keep on existinging.

Yet when there are numerous concepts, the possibilities of it spreading out rise; there are simply more individuals out there who are going to have the ability to gain access to it, discuss it, and undoubtedly, make it a part of their lives.

There are several kinds of yoga; and the reason for this, as we at first went over, is that yoga isn't a religion; it's a strategy to being alive. As such, it's really nimble and versatile and carries effectively throughout country, cultural, and religious borders.

Thanks to its variety and various aspects and types, yoga has actually spread out really promptly through the western world across the last 110 years or so; and is spreading out quicker now than ever prior (numerous western companies are now going to pay for yoga classes as potion of an improved health benefits program).

Yet this really variety has actually resulted in a bit of confusion; and individuals who have actually been exposed to one type of yoga may unintentionally believe that they've seen all of it. This is more worrisome, naturally, when one has actually been subjected to a type of yoga which-- for whichever reason-- they did not enjoy, or maybe, weren't rather prepared for (just as how some individuals may shy away from a fitness regimen if they aren't in the proper state of mind to persevere).

So if you have actually experienced yoga, or seen it on tv, read about it in a paper, or overheard a buddy or coworker speak about it, then please understand that there's a great chance that you have not been exposed to all that there is (and that is terrific, since it indicates that this following part is going to be really intriguing and helpful for you!).

6 Major Types

Yogic scholars Bodian and Feuerstein note 6 significant kinds of yoga. In no specific order, they are: Raja yoga, Hatha yoga, Bhakti yoga, Karma yoga, Jnana yoga, and Tantra yoga

Let's take a look at every one of these.

Hatha Yoga

Graham Ledgerwood, who has actually been instructing mysticism and yoga for over thirty years, states that hatha yoga is practiced in the west mainly for health and vigor, and is the most prominent in western world.

Ha is a Sanskrit word meaning sun, so hatha yoga, based upon Ledgerwood is a "magnificent means of working out, stretching, and releasing the body so it could be a long-lived, healthy, and essential instrument of the soul and mind.

Hatha yoga is considered as the 5000-year-old system that was utilized to boost the connection between body, spirit and mind. Individuals who do Hatha Yoga integrate the extending asanas exercises into their practice. It consists of psychological concentration and breathing methods.

The Lotus pose from Asanas is being utilized for practicing Hatha Yoga.

The objective of using Hatha Yoga is just the identical as utilizing other types of Yoga. It intends to mix the human spirit with the serene Universal spirit. With this practice, the individual performing the Yoga exercise boosts their spiritual, psychological, emotional and physical health.

Performing Hatha Yoga provides you with peace and maintains the world and your environment as one. In performing yoga, all kinds of yoga, concentration is the root or primary component for effective yoga.

All other kinds of Yoga have some resemblances in one way or the other. The primary aims of Hatha Yoga is to prep the body to give in so that the spirit is going to have the ability to absorb and achieve its objective. The spirit is accountable for raising and enlightening. When the spirit is enlightened, the mind is calmed and it gets rid of all stress and discomfort. The body does as well.

A lot of individuals get perplexed due to the fact that they do not comprehend that if your body is not fit and healthy; your spirit is not able to effectively accomplish the job. So Hatha Yoga is ideal to use in case your spirit is not strong.

Hatha Yoga is going to aid to motivate your body to move and advance favorably to a level where the spirit is going to have the ability to work correctly. Your body and spirit have to react favorably so that the mind can have the ability to keep up with an excellent concentration.

When individuals become aware of the word Yoga, Hatha Yoga is going pop in their minds initially. Hatha Yoga is well-known and it is the prominent Yoga branch. Actually, the other yoga styles like the Ashtanga, Kundalini, Bikram and Power Yoga actually stem from Hatha Yoga.

Hatha Yoga is considered as the vehicle for the soul. It is accountable for driving the spirit and the body into the universe. Simply picture skyrocketing to the universe without feeling any gravity whatsoever. That is so peaceful and appealing.

Concentration is a thing which is tough to sustain and recover. If you find yourself quickly sidetracked by external forces, Hatha Yoga may work to combat it.

The ideal feature of practicing Hatha Yoga is that it aids you to learn for your own that there is a divine light which shines in you. Not just does it enlighten you, yet it can aid you to end up being more powerful, unwinded and versatile.

The exercise associated with doing Hatha Yoga enables the spiritual energy to stream via the open energy channels. This is going to be feasible if the mind, spirit and body are working great. Obviously, preserving a healthy body is the most essential of all. If your body is not strong, your spirit and mind are impacted as well.

As you practice Hatha Yoga, you could quickly cope with tension and alleviate some discomfort and stress. Often, work leaves you drained and tired so you want to unwind from time to time. Hatha Yoga is the ideal solution to discharge that discomfort and stress.

Refining the poses in hatha yoga has 2 goals:

1. Meditating.

Individuals require at least one posture which they are able to be completely comfy with, for an extended time period. The more poses you are able to master, the more you are able to cultivate better meditation methods.

2. Restoring the body's energies for optimal health.

Raja Yoga

Comparable to classical yoga, Raja Yoga is seen as the "royal path" to unifying the body and mind. Raja yoga is thought about by some to be a rather challenging type of yoga since it looks for enlightenment via straight control and competence of the mind.

Individuals who can focus effectivelly and delight in meditation are ideally suited for Raja yoga. This kind of yoga has 8 limbs: Moral discipline, posture, self-restraint, sensory inhibition, breath control, meditation, concentration, and ecstasy.

Karma Yoga

Karma yoga features selfless action. The word karma itself indicates action-- all action which originates from the individual starts from his birth up until his end. Most notably, karma is the road to doing the appropriate thing. For this reason, the karma yoga practice suggests renouncing on the ego to serve God and humankind.

Karma yoga originates from the Bhagavad Vita teachings, which is often respectfully described as "the Hindu New Testament ." Service to God via serving others is the groundwork of Karma Yoga.

Bhakti Yoga

In this kind of highest Bhakti, all attachment and attraction that someone has for things of satisfaction are moved to the sole dearest object, God. This guides the followers to an everlasting union with his Beloved and results in in oneness."

Bhakti yoga is therefore viewed as magnificent love. As a force of attraction, Sri Ramakrishna Math and Swami Nikhilananda state that love functions on 3 levels: Material, spiritual and human.

These 2 yogis additionally clarify that love is a creative power, and this power drives us to look for happiness and immortality. In their own sophisticated and exact words:

Love based upon intellectual attraction is more impersonal and lasting. It is a question of common observation which the more intellectually established the life of an individual is, the less he gets a kick out of the things of the senses.

Jnana Yoga

Jnana yoga is the road to wisdom. Graham Ledgerwood specifies jnana as "emptying" the mind and soul of misconceptions so that people could be attuned to truth, releasing all ideas and feelings up until the person is enlightened and transformed.

Jnana yoga is among the 4 primary paths which lead straight to self-realization. By squashing the barriers of ignorance, the trainee of jnana yoga experiences God.

Ideas like discrimination and discernment are extremely regarded in Jnana yoga, where the trainee or devotee recognizes himself as separate from the parts of his environment. "Neti-neti" is likewise a concept inherent in Jnana Yoga. Actually, it means "not this, not this" and by getting rid of the things around, what remains is simply YOU and just you.

Tantra Yoga.

The last kind of yoga which numerous individuals have actually heard about, and undoubtedly, are rather intrigued by, is tantra yoga.

Tantra yoga is thought about by some folks to be most oriental of all branches of yoga. It is frequently misinterpreted as consisting solely of sexual routines. It includes more than sex: it is the road of self-transcendence via ritual means, among which is simply consecrated sexuality. Certain tantric schools really suggest a celibate way of life after a specific point.

Tantra actually means "expansion." A Tantra devotee broadens all his levels of awareness so that person could connect to the Supreme Truth. Tantra yoga intends to awaken the female and male elements within an individual to set off a spiritual awakening.

Tantra yoga is more focused on spiritual healing, and most importantly, the integration of the mind, body, and spirit. In India, it is an ancient custom that sexuality is an essential and substantial stage to be able to attain a particular level of enlightenment.

In Western religious norms, sexual gratifications and desires are not inclined or connected with spirituality. With these distinctions in customs, there is a fine line between their feelings and perspectives towards sexuality together with spirituality.

Nevertheless, in Eastern philosophy, they rejoice and celebrate the elegance and magnificence of creation. And further on, they have actually established a science or study for comprehending how to get most of this restorative and terrific experience. Energy is recognized to be the life source in Tantra.

Moreover, they think about sexual energy and desire as fantastic and spiritual energy. There are a few of the numerous exercises which assist in the performance of the sexual element along with certain dietary changes. A few of these physical exercises consist of contractions, breathing and holding particular poses.

There are a lot of advantages which could be acquired by carrying out these different physical exercises. A few of these entail enhanced prostate functioning and better and enhanced sexual performance. Another advantage is enhanced sexual endurance when taking part in sexual intercourse.

There are likewise various types of exercises. Beside the physical exercises, there are psycho-spiritual workouts. These exercises are methods to establish mediation on desire and unconditional love. Consequently, this could make sexual activities less uncomfortable and anxious, aside from that, the pressure to execute and move is decreased.

It is stated that the most remarkable sexual experience is giving in entirely to your lover or partner what that person actually desires. Expectations might be high, so one needs to perform.

Through meditation and correct exercises, one can think of the numerous manners in which he could please his lover. When one is concentrated and focused on offering what the lover truly desires is an experience that can reinforce the relationship with one another, you are going to get the satisfaction you had actually always desired. There are a couple of exercises that could assist you a lot with concentrating on your sexual performance.

By repeating certain chants and mantras along with breathing exercises and appropriate meditation, one could attain these advantages.

There are likewise many methods to take your foreplay to the utmost level. With healing massages and mild stroking, one could get a gratifying experience which promote both spiritual and physical healing in various ways.

Reiki or energy channeling healing is engaged in prior to taking part in sexual activity. This is recognized to elevate sexual enjoyment in intercourse. It is an Eastern healing art where one partner channels his energy to the other.

Via tactile stimulation, healing is attained and both the spiritual and physical element are boosted. In this way, both of you can attain a much deeper state of meditation and relaxation that is extremely useful to partnerships and couples.

Advice for Novices

As you now understand, yoga is an extremely intriguing and ancient method of unifying the mind and body. It has actually proven health advantages, featuring psychological and physical improvements.

The chances for that reason are, if you're on the brink of beginning a yoga program (possibly at a neighborhood center or you have actually bought a DVD or video and wish to try it in your home), you're delighted, positive, and anxious to start!

Yet it's smart to keep in mind that, prior to entering into yoga practice, you must ask yourself certain essential questions. These questions do not have a correct or incorrect response.

They are simply supposed to stimulate your own ideas and provide you with the state of mind that you require so as to prosper as a trainee of yoga for the long run.

Here are the fundamental questions which you ought to ask prior to beginning any yoga program:

What are my reasons for beginning a yoga program? Are they reasonable?

If my yoga program includes certain level of physical stress, like specific poses in hatha yoga, have I received medical clearance from a certified and licensed health expert to make sure that I do not hurt myself?

Are my objectives for going after a yoga program positive and clear? Do I understand what I wish to attain?

Am I ready to devote the time needed to actually get the most out of my yoga experience?

Are there individuals around me who may adversely try to talk me out (or mock me out) of pursuing this course of personal growth? Should I either stay away from such individuals or ask them to respect what I want to do?

Please keep in mind that these are simply fundamental questions, and this isn't an extensive list. The point here is truly that you ought to be clear and positive about your choice of experiencing yoga.

And keep in mind, please: there are various types of yoga and various types of instructors. The majority of them are excellent; a handful of them might be well-intentioned, yet might lack a few of the foundations which they require so as to teach.

Keep in mind: no yoga instructor which you deal with should ever embarrass you, insult you, degrade you, or make you feel inferior.

If you come across the one in a thousand who has actually not yet attained the personal growth that he/she requires so as to teach successfully, then keep in mind: there are always other instructors!

The objective here is to make you delighted, healthy, and positive. These requirements ought to be a portion of all of your yoga experiences from the first day.

One More Thing about Consistency

For you to delight in each benefit of your dedication to practicing yoga, please keep in mind that regularity and consistency are keys. You can't enter into one session and miss 3 or 4 even if you're sore, had an unanticipated engagement, or are too stressed.

For the mind and body to alter, you have to practice yoga regularly. Eliminate all barriers, imagined or real and remain devoted. Your benefits are going to be much better health, much better psychological balance, and a more fulfilled, happier life!

Chapter 4: Yoga Positions

Yoga positions for novices are rather simple to learn. If you have actually not experienced any yoga session or have actually not seen one, that is not an issue.

Professionals have spoken about the unification of the body, mind and spirit. They declared that this is going to be obtained via the practice of yoga exercises and methods.

If it is your initial time you hear of yoga, you are going to, naturally, question how these exercises are performed and what it looks like. Given that you are a novice, you are going to certainly ask what positions are going to be ideal for you.

Yogis have believed that the body and the mind are bound into a unified structure. This belief has actually never ever falled short and altered across time. Yoga has thoroughly performed an incredible procedure of recovering oneself via harmony. This could be effectively accomplished if you are in an appropriate environment.

With the fantastic impacts of yoga, medical professionals have actually been convinced that yoga has some restorative outcomes and that it can be advised for individuals who have health problems that are difficult to treat.

If you have some health problem which has been with you for a long period of time, you could practice the yoga poses for novices and apply it to yourself.

If you wish to practice the yoga poses for newbies, you need to trust that yoga works and is going to aid you to be healed or be revitalized.

Yoga is not simply a recent application. It has actually been practiced and used a very long time ago and individuals are still benefitting from it.

Examinations have been carried out to show that yoga could be useful in the recovery process.

For that reason, it has actually been shown that yoga poses for newbies are incredibly helpful and beneficial when it pertains to preserving a high degree of joint flexibility. Even though the yoga poses for newbies are just basic and simple, it can gradually bring up a healthy way of life when it is practiced repeatedly.

The yoga poses for newbies are extremely intriguing and amazing to carry out. Beginners are never going to find it tough to keep up with the exercises since it is just simple. The yoga technique provides a huge contributing element to our internal organs and glands. It likewise consists of the parts of the body that are rarely stimulated.

If you wish to find out yoga positions for newbies, you could discover it simply at home or at school where yoga is instructed.

Some standard yoga poses for novices consist of standing postures, seated postures, backward and forward bends, twisting and balance.

The time duration in carrying out the positions is likewise reduced since a novice can not totally deal with long-time exposure in practice. Rest is needed by the novice so that he is not going to be drained easily to prep the body for additional positions.

If you are a newbie, the most essential thing you ought to have is self-discipline. Yoga is not simply doing yoga and carrying out the positions. If you have not mastered the fundamentals yet, do not delve into the complex phases and positions since you are not going to feel the essence of carrying out the yoga positions for novices.

Managing Yoga positions.

There are a great deal of yoga positions and postures which are developed to enhance posture.

Yoga positions have a great deal of benefits like enhancing our posture and providing us with a straight figure.

Often, we may find our selves in an uneven figure. If we practice that for a very long time without doing anything about it, expect to have a misaligned bone in the future.

Yoga poses are excellent to reinforce our body providing focus to the knces, thighs and the ankles. If you get accustomed to practicing yoga poses daily, it is expected that your bones react instantly.

The abdominal area and the buttocks are seen as a significant turn-on for both genders. For the male, it is best to maintain a great abdominal area. This makes it more attractive to ladies.

Having an excellent butt matters to certain women as well, a great deal of them are practicing so as to shape their bodies nicely.

Yoga positions incredibly alleviate sciatica. These are certain pains which can not be prevented. If you do yoga occasionally and even routinely, perhaps you are not going to feel any muscle or back discomfort.

Here are certain methods on how to maintain an excellent yoga pose. Simply follow these steps so as to completely understand yoga poses and have the ability to perform them in the correct manner.

1. You need to stand with the bases of your big toes touching and the heels ought to be somewhat apart. You need to raise and spread your toes gradually and the balls of your feet as well. Then after, you have to lay them gently down on the floor. Rock yourself backward and forward and even side to side. You might slowly lower this swaying to preserve a standstill, with your weight balanced uniformly on your feet.

2. Harden your thigh muscles, and after that, raise the knee caps. Do it without hardening the lower belly. Raise the inner ankles to create more powerful internal arches, then imagine a line of energy all the way up along your inner thighs up to your groin area. From there through the core of your neck, head, and torso, and out through the crown of your head. You ought to turn the upper thighs gradually inward. Make your tailbone longer

toward the ground and raise the pubis in the navel's direction.

3. Press your shoulder blades into your back, then expand them crossways and release them down your back. Without roughly pressing your lower front ribs forward, raise the top of your sternum directly towards the ceiling. Expand your collarbones. Suspend your arms alongside the torso.

4. You ought to balance the crown of your head unswervingly over the pelvis middle, with your chin's base analogous to the ground, soft throat, and the broad tongue and plane on your mouth's floor. Make your eyes appear softer.

5. Tadasana is generally the first yoga pose for all the standing postures. Using Tansana works particularly in applying the positions. Remain in the posture for 30 seconds up to 1 minute, then breathe easily to keep it satisfying.

Simply follow these basic figures so that you can be certain that you are performing everything appropriately.

Strike it up With Your Yoga Postures

There are a great deal of yoga postures and you may question if some are still done and used. The response is yes. Yoga postures perform and function differently. Each position is created to establish one's strength and flexibility.

Here are a few of the yoga positions which are typically utilized:

Standing Positions

Standing is among the essential yoga postures. This kind of position is useful in aligning your feet and body. This is likewise extremely helpful in enhancing and preserving an excellent posture. It is an advantage since if you have a bad posture, your backbones could be extended and aligned without seeing it. Standing positions help in providing strength to your legs and at the identical time increasing flexibility in your hips and legs due to the fact that they are all linked to one another.

Seated Positions.

These kinds of yoga postures boost your hip and lower back flexibility. This likewise reinforces your back. This includes flexibility to your groin, knees, ankle and, most particularly, your spinal column. Another benefit is that it aids you to breathe in deeply which provides you that calm and serene sensation.

Forward Bends

This type assists you in stretching your lower back and the hamstrings, additionally strengthening it. This minimizes the tension discovered in your shoulder, neck, back and increases flexibility in your spinal column. Calmness is likewise attained in this kind of position.

Back bends are exceptionally useful in opening your hips, chest and even the rib cage. This is useful in fortifying and making your shoulders and arms more powerful. At the identical time, it simultaneously boosts elasticity and flexibility in your shoulders. The terrific thing is that it aids to ease the tension from your body's front up to your hips and it boost your spinal capability. Your spine is something that is essential to your body so you want to take excellent care of it.

Back Bends

Notice that the forward bends are tough since the exercise offers you a great sensation and it could lead you to repair certain injuries. In this kind of position, you could utilize a prop such as a strap or black due to the fact that it is going to be extremely useful.

Balance

Balance positions are really difficult. Individuals who do yoga get too fired up about carrying out balances. This is excellent due to the fact that the fun that the individual gets aids him to enlighten his soul and liven up his spirit. Balance is valuable in enhancing your posture. In enhancing your posture, the spine is lengthened which aids to protect yourself from certain injuries and tipping over.

Balance aids in training your capability to concentrate on your primary goal and attention. Nevertheless, attention must be acquired at the supreme level due to the fact that if your focus is not strong, you can not carry out this kind of posture.

Balance is one of the yoga postures which individuals really value and put in the effort for. Along with the balance positions comes the twist that exceptionally releases tension all across your body. The tension in your spinal column is made apparent. Twisting might appear to be tough to perform. It is essential to carry out twists on both sides to ensure that the alignment and balance are acquired.

Taking note of these yoga positions is going to aid you to get along with yoga completely. Remember that concentration is your primary key if you wish to achieve success in performing these yoga postures.

Chapter 5: Tool & Accessories for Yoga

The appeal of yoga has actually produced a market which specializes in yoga equipment, accessories and clothing. The web is a real market place of things that are related to yoga and product lines are as diverse and varied as the numerous teachings and positions of yoga.

If you have actually gone into your neighborhood sporting shop and even a department shop, you've most likely seen a variety of yoga equipment which features really pleased and serene looking individuals resting on a yoga mat, or utilizing a yoga towel. Undoubtedly, for somebody thinking about yoga, this is akin to a kid in a candy store. There has never ever been a time in the market where yoga equipment was so simple to discover, and undoubtedly, so budget-friendly!

With that being stated, it could be rather complicated as to which equipment does what. They all appear to have such delighted looking individuals on the packaging; how do you know what deserves your cash?

Well, eventually, the response to that crucial question is going to be identified by the sort of yoga which you wish to experience, and likewise, your own preferences.

Certain individuals, for instance, do not wish to rest on a mat; they prefer the firmness of the ground. Other individuals find that resting on the ground hurts and could result in tailbone and back ache; and as such, a yoga mat is vital.

So, instead of recommending here what you ought to purchase and what you must not, let's rather concentrate on the numerous cool things that you can quickly purchase, and you could utilize this information to aid you to make a smart decision.

Yoga Mats

Let's begin with the popular yoga mat. Now, as a basic guideline: be careful with the supermarket model.

A great yoga mat has a great grip on the floor, which is essential if you need to carry out complex postures and maneuvers. They generally measure about 2 feet in width, and are offered in a multitude of rainbow colors.

There are yoga mats to fit all levels from newbie to advanced, and you have a selection of thickness. Lots of yoga shops are going to supply mats with effective cushioning. Yoga mats are likewise offered for kids.

Yoga Towel

Do not forget your yoga towel. There are additionally skidless towels and certain producers create very absorbent ones-- also, in what certain retailers refer to as "chakra colors."

Yoga Bags

Yoga bags appear rectangular-- nearly tubular-- they are developed to hold your towel and yoga mat and other accessories.

A lot of products have a shoulder strap and are created from various materials, nylon being a typical one. There are low-end yoga bags retailing for $13.00 and they go up to $50.00, based upon how it is made and its size.

Yoga Straps

Those who do a great deal of flexibility routines frequently choose yoga straps. These straps aid them to stretch their limbs, and to hold postures for more time.

Yoga Bolsters and Sandbags

There are additionally yoga bolsters and sandbags which aid your body balance and supply support as you carry out your postures, positions and stretches. They are additionally offered in numerous colors.

Yoga Balls

Balls are great for developing strength, attaining balance and toning muscles. These enjoyable yoga balls cost about $25.00, and numerous dancers and physiotherapists utilize yoga balls for a range of motions, consisting of backbends, corrective positions, and hip openers. Lots of balls can hold up to 600 pounds.

Yoga Blocks

These tools appear like blocks and feel like a mattress. They're terrific for body movement extensions.

Yoga Videos/DVDs

If you're starved for time, feel a tad shy about participating in a public yoga class, or simply wish to have a clue about how yoga is practiced, yoga DVDs/videos are an excellent method to get started with yoga.

A fantastic benefit of yoga videos is you can see the clips repeatedly up until you have actually mastered the methods properly.

Yoga Music

Think about trying yoga music to aid you to practice meditation better, breathe deeper, and hold those poses for more time.

To name a couple of titles: Tibetan Sacred Temple Music, Slow Music for Yoga, Nectar, Shiva Station, Fragrance of the East, and so on.

There is even yoga music for yoga flow and trance dance, mantras and chants and audiobooks.

Yoga Clothes

Though not necessary for class, lots of yoga participants desire all-yoga outfit to match their yoga practice. A lot of newbies, nevertheless, come in a loose-fitting cotton t-shirt and comfy leggings.

In picking the ideal yoga clothing, obviously, they ought to be comfy and created to provide you a relaxing effect.

The ideal yoga clothes are those which enable you to easily move and protect against instances of interruption and disruption when you are having your practice. They have to feel excellent on your skin so that you are going to be devoid from tenderness.

Yoga clothing is a crucial accessory since it sets you into the proper state of mind. If you do not have the ideal set of yoga clothing, your practicing day is not going to be great.

Throughout a heavy practice, it is anticipated that you are going to sweat excessively. Some individuals do not actually sweat too much; however, if you do, you ought to wear absorbent clothing to ensure that the sweat is going to be lessened, offering you a dry sensation.

When you are all covered by sweat, you are going to have that sticky feeling that maintains you uneasy and in some cases, scratchy.

Even though yoga clothing does not have to look that great, it is still crucial that you wear appealing ones so that you are going to have a great feel and look. Self-confidence is, likewise, an impacting factor in practicing. If you wear excellent yoga clothes, then you are not going to feel discriminated. So pick the ideal clothes which are going to match with your character.

In practicing yoga, there is no need in picking your clothes. If you wish to display some skin, it depends on you. If your body has a good shape, you can wear fitting t-shirts and trousers.

If you do not have that figure and believe that you have the guts, nobody is going to scold you. Besides, you're the one who carries your body as long as you are able to manage it.

Here are the typical things you require when searching for yoga clothes.

1. Yoga Tops-- the initial thing you ought to think about in selecting a yoga top is that it must not fall in your face. Tops are created to allow you to move freely and not be sidetracked when performing the exercise. If you will wear tee-shirts, it must not be that long and must not cover the lower part of your body. This is necessary in checking the positioning of your lower body due to the fact that you can see whether your ankles and knees are lined up correctly. Many ladies use sports bras so that in performing certain motions, they are certain that it holds them firmly.

2. Yoga Pants-- Picking your yoga pants is rather delicate. The surface and texture of certain trousers might not offer you a comfy feel. The length of the trousers is among the important things to think about in picking them. Some trousers are so long that they reach your ankles. If this is not comfy for you, you should wear trousers which are below your knees. This enables you to move easily.

3. Yoga Shorts-- this is an excellent option if you are practicing hot yoga, or otherwise called, Bikram Yoga. This kind of yoga is carried out in a room at a high temperature. Wearing shorts is going to release the heat within your body.

Selecting your yoga clothes does not suggest that it needs to be costly. What is necessary is that you feel great and comfy deep within.

Conclusion

The yoga journey is one which is constantly an introduction. There is no conclusion of yoga; it is a continuous procedure of finding yourself and stimulating your body to provide it with ideal health.

Among other things, this guide has preferably:

Shown you that yoga is not a religion and for that reason, does not request or demand from you to alter your faith.

Assisted you in comprehending the advantages of yoga; advantages that vary from physical, to psychological, to mental improvements.

Assisted you to comprehend that yoga is not an "overnight thing," but requires consistency, dedication, and routine so as to provide all of the advantages which you are worthy of.

Assisted you to comprehend the numerous different types of yoga out there (and all of these types are available in the west, via a few of the less prominent ones may only be centered in big metropolitan locations).

Supplied you with an overview of the different equipment which you could acquire (if you want!) to improve and enhance your journey.

I hope that you enjoyed reading through this book and that you have found it useful. If you want to share your thoughts on this book, you can do so by leaving a review on the Amazon page. Have a great rest of the day.

Printed in Great Britain
by Amazon

46478366R00047